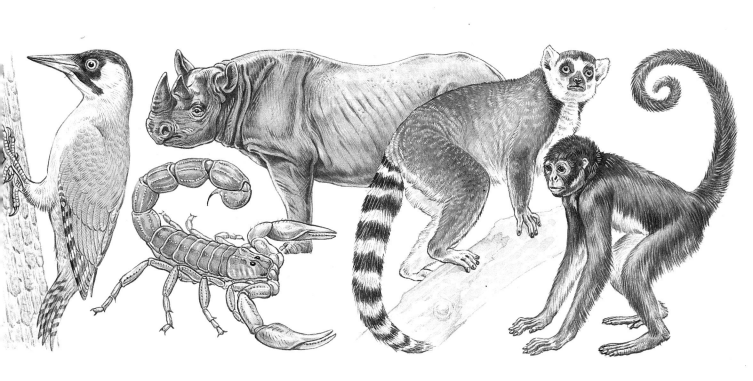

Contents

Illustrators:

Steve Burgess pages 8-9

John Butler pages 36-37

Barbara Firth pages 12-13, 14-15

Gerrard McIvor pages 40-41, 42-43

Dee Morgan pages 16-17, 32-33, 38-39

George Sharp pages 6-7, 10-11

Peter Snowball pages 44-45, end sheets, title page, cover

Peter Visscher pages 26-27, 34-35

David Wright pages 18-19, 20-21, 22-23, 24-25, 28-29, 30-31

Editor: David Lloyd

Art editor: Pat Butterworth

Consultants: Cuillin Bantock
            Louise Gordon
            Chris Humphreys

First American edition published in 1984 by
Peter Bedrick Books
125 East 23 Street
New York, N.Y. 10010

Published by agreement with Walker Books Ltd., London.

Library of Congress Cataloguing in Publication Data
Freeman, Dan.
  Beautiful bodies.
  Includes index.
  Summary: Explains the composition and workings of all the parts of the human body.
  1. Body, Human – Juvenile literature. [1. Body, human 2. Physiology] I. Title.
QP37.F67 1984 612 83-25723
ISBN 0-911745-52-1

Manufactured in Italy
Distributed in the USA by Harper & Row

The world is so full of a number of things,
I'm sure we should all be as happy as kings.

Robert Louis Stevenson

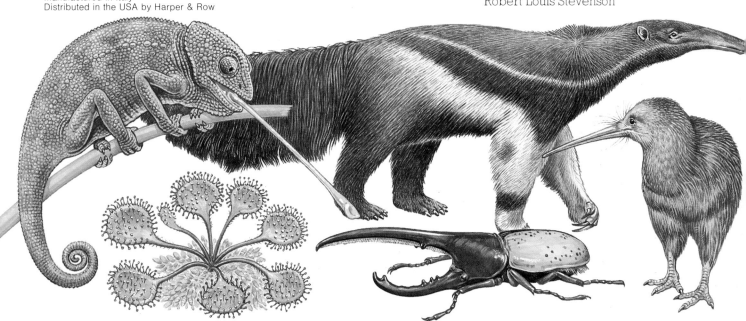

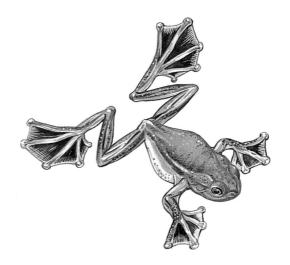

BEAUTIFUL BODIES

Written by Dan Freeman

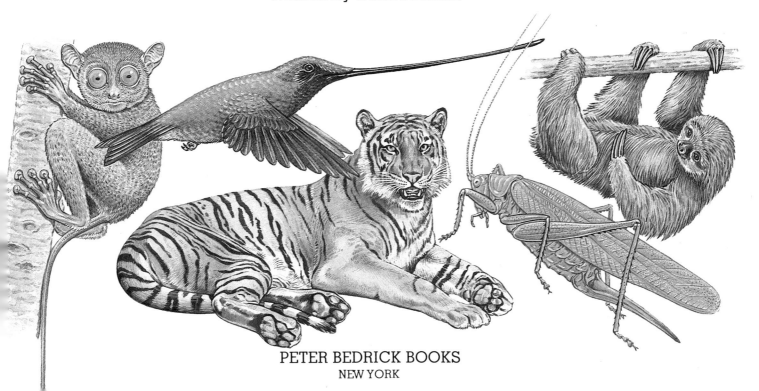

PETER BEDRICK BOOKS
NEW YORK

Body work

A body is somewhere to live – a home designed through millions of years of evolution, a place that is different every day of its life. A body works, and in its working you come alive. When your body is well, you enjoy it. When it is hurt, you nurse it. Every day you feed, exercise and rest it. In its inner ways of working it is more complicated than you may ever understand. It has circuits and systems more intricate than those of any computer. But its basic needs are relatively few. If these are satisfied your body may keep going for 100 years or more.

Under your skin work is always going on at a tremendous pace. The brain issues as many as 100 million orders every second: messages flash out, every part of you responds in its special way. Day or night there is no end to the work, as more than 20,000 million nerve cells protect your life. Your heart beats, your lungs breathe, all the hidden organs of your body perform their essential tasks. As you lie in bed, play in the sun or walk down the street, all this happens without your needing to give it any thought. In numberless ways your body keeps its work a secret.

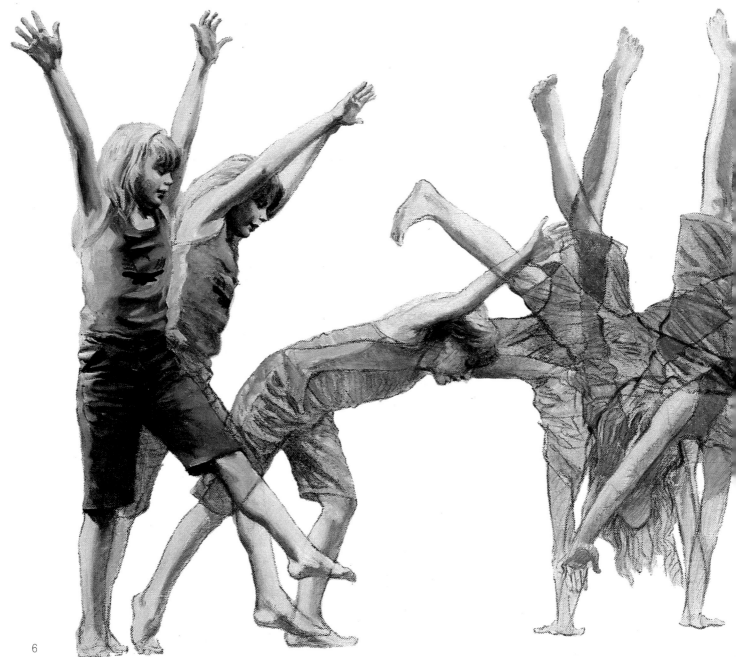

Even when you are sitting still, your body uses up a great deal of energy just staying alive. It cannot make energy out of nothing. It needs fuel, as a car needs petrol, and it gets it from food. The body hungers, so you feed it. Hunger is the body's way of calling attention to its need for fuel.

With your teeth you chew the food, with your tongue you stir it, with your saliva you help to liquefy it. When you swallow, the food enters a pathway through your body, which is about 8m long in an adult. Here some 20 different chemical substances break it down into its simple components, such as fats, carbohydrates and proteins. These enter your blood, are inspected and purified by your liver, and are carried all over you by your bloodstream. The whole process takes about six hours. Then you start to feel hungry again.

You are made of food, you grow out of food, you live on food. This is the pleasure of eating. Life enters you with every meal you take, building your body from inside. Take a bite from an apple. The taste on your tongue is energy, as the apple goes to work for you.

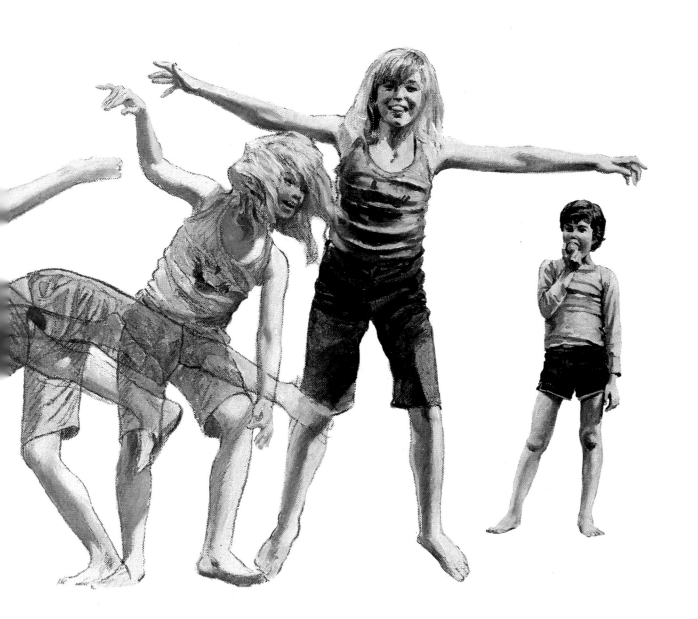

Under your skin

In your hand there are 27 bones, so neatly jointed that they can pick, point, hold, grasp, wave, beckon and perform thousands of other precise or powerful movements. Without them your hand would be floppy, feeble and useless. In your head there are 29 bones. Eight of them can move slightly at birth, but soon lock rigidly together to shield your brain. A further 14 make up your face. Deep in your ears are the smallest bones in your body, about 3mm long, which help pass sounds to your brain. Your lower jaw is the only bone in your head which can move freely. Altogether more than 200 separate bones give your body its shape, protect the most important organs inside it and, working with your muscles, enable you to move however you like.

From a third to a half of the weight of your body is muscle, the powerpack where energy is stored and released on demand. Some muscles move bones, contracting to pull them up like levers, relaxing to let others pull them down again. Others, like the ones which move food through your body, work automatically, without your needing to think about them. When you smile, you work 17 muscles. When you frown, you work 43. Your body

Muscle

Some 650 muscles make the meat of your body, accounting for over a third of your weight. Muscles move your bones by pulling them, never by pushing. When you bend your arm, muscles pull it up. When you straighten it, others muscles pull it down again.

Skeleton

Your bones account for about a fifth of the weight of your body. An adult has 206 bones, a baby some 300 – some of the bones join together as you grow up. The strongest bone in your body is your thigh bone – when a pole-vaulter lands, it takes an impact of more than three-quarters of a tonne per square centimetre.

has some 650 muscles in all, mostly arranged in small groups. If they were made into one pair of gigantic muscles working one giant set of bones, they would be strong enough to lift three large elephants.

Your heart is an organ about the size of your clenched fist, made almost entirely of muscle. It is the pump which drives blood through your body, delivering food needed for energy to all your cells. One of the most important journeys blood makes is to your brain. If your brain is deprived of the oxygen in blood for more than three minutes, it suffers permanent damage. So its message to the heart is simple. Keep on beating – 72 times a minute, nearly 5,000 times an hour, 750,000 times a week. If you live until you are 100, it will have worked hard enough to fill a vessel with a capacity of more than 250 million litres.

There are about five litres of blood in your body, transporting their cargo through a web of tubes – veins, arteries and capillaries – some 160,000 km long. Here, too, special cells patrol your body, ready to attack any germs or other invaders which could make you ill. Curiously, the substance on earth which most closely resembles blood is sea-water – where most people think that life began.

Heart and blood
Some five litres of blood, pumped by the never-resting muscles of your heart, flow continuously through the 160,000 km or so of veins, arteries and capillaries in your body. They take life-giving substances to all your cells, clear out their waste, and fight any disease which threatens to make you ill.

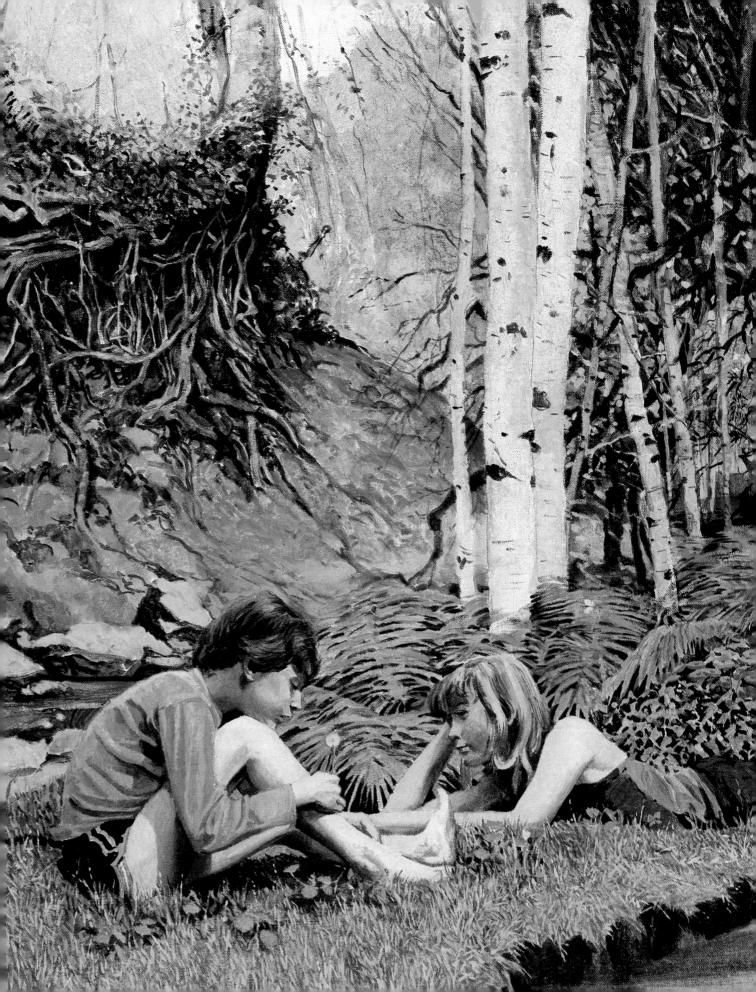

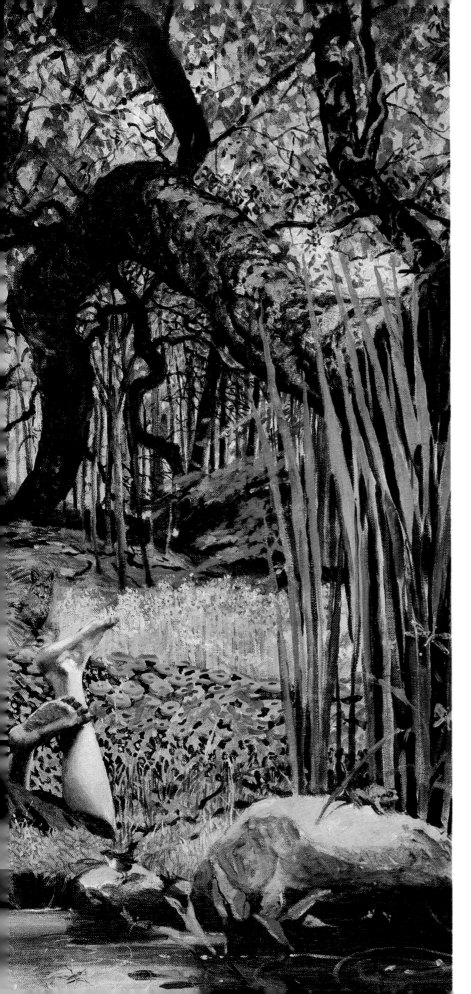

The dandelion and you

Your arms and legs, your bones and muscles, your heart, nerves and blood – every part of you is made of cells, the building blocks of life. Each cell has a life of its own. Every second millions of cells are born in your body, and millions of others die. You grow as your cells multiply. Your body also keeps itself new, as fresh cells replace worn-out ones. Even your bones are alive. New bone cells replace old ones so fast that in less than two years your skeleton changes completely.

All bodies in the world are made of cells – your body, the body of every living animal, the roots, stem, leaves and all other parts of all plants' bodies. Animals and plants may seem quite different, but really they are very alike. They are both made of cells. They are both small to start with and grow up. They both have offspring. They both feed. Plants even share with animals the ability to move. A flower's petals open and close, a pea plant reaches out tendrils like arms, leaves turn towards the sun.

Plants and animals live together in a sort of marriage. Plants use carbon dioxide from the air, and water and sunlight to make sugars for energy. They give out oxygen. Animals use the oxygen and eat plants or other animals to make their energy. They give out carbon dioxide. Plants use the carbon dioxide. If there were no plants, there could be no animals either.

The world can support as much life as it does because of this sort of organisation. If all bodies needed the same things at the same time, the result would be chaos. As it is, life exists in balance, because all species are adapted to survive in different ways. Each lives in its own way, according to the design of its body. You and a dandelion are different so that both of you can live together in the same world.

The important thing is life itself. Adaptation makes all the differences between bodies and ways of life. But life is the same for all – for you and the dandelion, for all the living bodies on earth.

Standing still

A tree looks very still, standing in the sun on a summer's day. But looks are deceptive. Under its bark all sorts of movements are going on, just as they are under your skin. Great quantities of mineral-rich water are rising from its roots to its leaves – as many as 400 litres a day in a well-grown tree. Every leaf is hard at work, making sugars to feed the tree. The sugars travel back through the tree in a liquid called sap, nourishing the tree in all its parts and helping it to grow. A tree keeps growing all its life, quickly in summer, hardly at all in winter.

In the green of a leaf lies the key to how plants live. The green is a pigment called chlorophyll, which stores energy from sunlight. Every leaf is a chemical workshop, where water reacts with carbon dioxide from the air to make sugars. The sun's energy stored in chlorophyll provides the power for the workshop. Plants have no need to go looking for food, as animals must. They can make food wherever they are.

A plant stands still for all its life, rooted in the soil where it first fell as a seed. But to produce seeds itself, it must reach beyond itself to breed with another of its own species. The flower which blooms on a plant is one way of doing this. Flowers have male parts called stamens, and female ovaries. Pollen from the stamens – sometimes carried by insects and sometimes by the wind – fertilizes female cells in the ovaries. Then the fertilized flowers grow into seeds.

Plants have evolved many ways of distributing their seeds. Some seeds float on the wind, some are dispersed by streams or rain. In some species, like gorse, the fruit explodes, catapulting the seeds away from the parent plant. In many, animals scatter the seeds – getting them accidently caught on their fur, storing nuts in places where eventually they germinate, or eating the fruit and later excreting the seeds unharmed. These are some of the ways in which plants move, though their bodies must always stand still.

Oak tree

Skeleton of wood

A tree's trunk and branches are alive. Like a skeleton, they give the tree its shape, enabling it to hold its leaves up to the sun. Just under the protective bark, water flows continuously upwards from the roots, and sugary sap – the tree's lifeblood – flows back from the leaves.

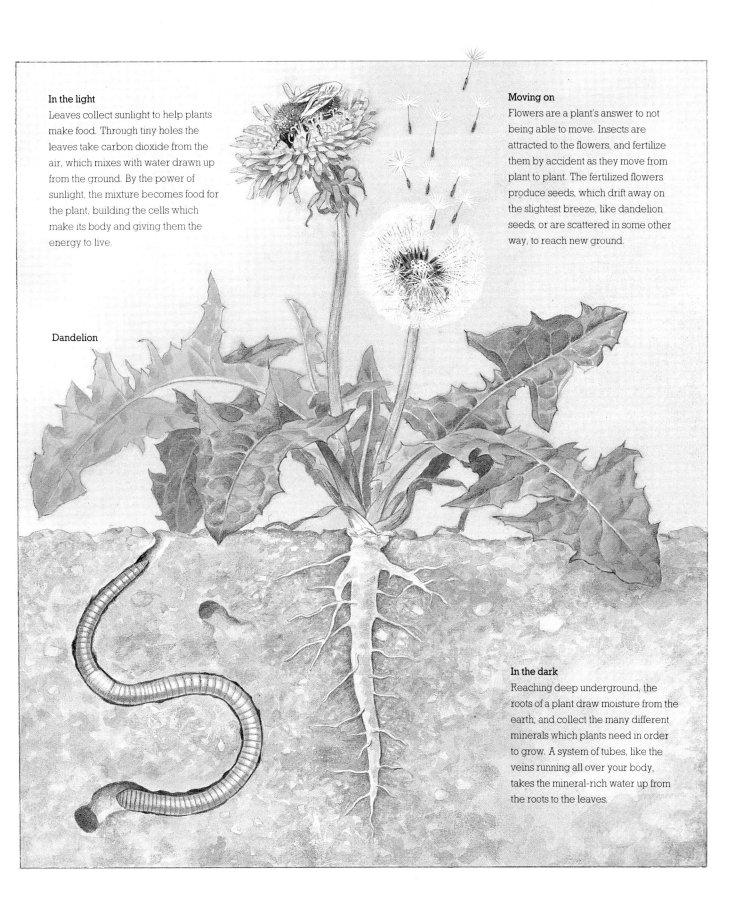

In the light

Leaves collect sunlight to help plants make food. Through tiny holes the leaves take carbon dioxide from the air, which mixes with water drawn up from the ground. By the power of sunlight, the mixture becomes food for the plant, building the cells which make its body and giving them the energy to live.

Moving on

Flowers are a plant's answer to not being able to move. Insects are attracted to the flowers, and fertilize them by accident as they move from plant to plant. The fertilized flowers produce seeds, which drift away on the slightest breeze, like dandelion seeds, or are scattered in some other way, to reach new ground.

Dandelion

In the dark

Reaching deep underground, the roots of a plant draw moisture from the earth, and collect the many different minerals which plants need in order to grow. A system of tubes, like the veins running all over your body, takes the mineral-rich water up from the roots to the leaves.

The wildest garden

Single cells floating in the sea, containing chlorophyll to trap sunlight, were probably among the earliest forms of life on earth. These were the first plants. After millions of years their descendants colonised the land. They evolved roots to find the moisture in soil, and stems to help them reach towards the sun. They spread across the earth, and their bodies adapted in countless ways to the conditions around them. Animal life has always depended on them. The success story of plants is evident not just in the number of plants on earth, but also in their variety. So far some 300,000 species of plants have been named, and thousands more join the list every year. From the simplest seed the wildest garden grew, raised by the energy of the sun.

Life in the water
In order to grow in still water or slow-moving rivers, water lilies have long, trailing roots which anchor them to the bottom. Their leaves are big, because they gather sunlight on only one side, and spongy so that they float. At night the flowers close, and sometimes sink below the surface until morning comes.

Life underground
The permanent, ageing part of a daffodil lives underground. In spring the underground bulb sends up leaves to gather sunlight. Then a flower grows, attracting insects to help the plant breed. When the flower dies and seeds have been produced, the leaves stay alive for a few months more, making food to be stored in the bulb.

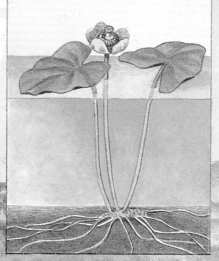

In heat and drought
Cacti can survive intense heat and lack of rain, which would quickly kill most plants. They have swollen, fleshy stems, which store as much water as possible, and tough skin through which little water is lost. Their leaves are sharp spines which also lose little water, and protect the plants from thirsty animals.

Waiting in the dust
The seeds of Sturt's desert pea may lie for ten years in the dry, red dust of the Australian outback. When a rainstorm finally comes, the water washes a protective coating from the seed. In a brief, brilliant lifetime, the plant grows, flowers and produces new seeds, which lie waiting once more in the dust.

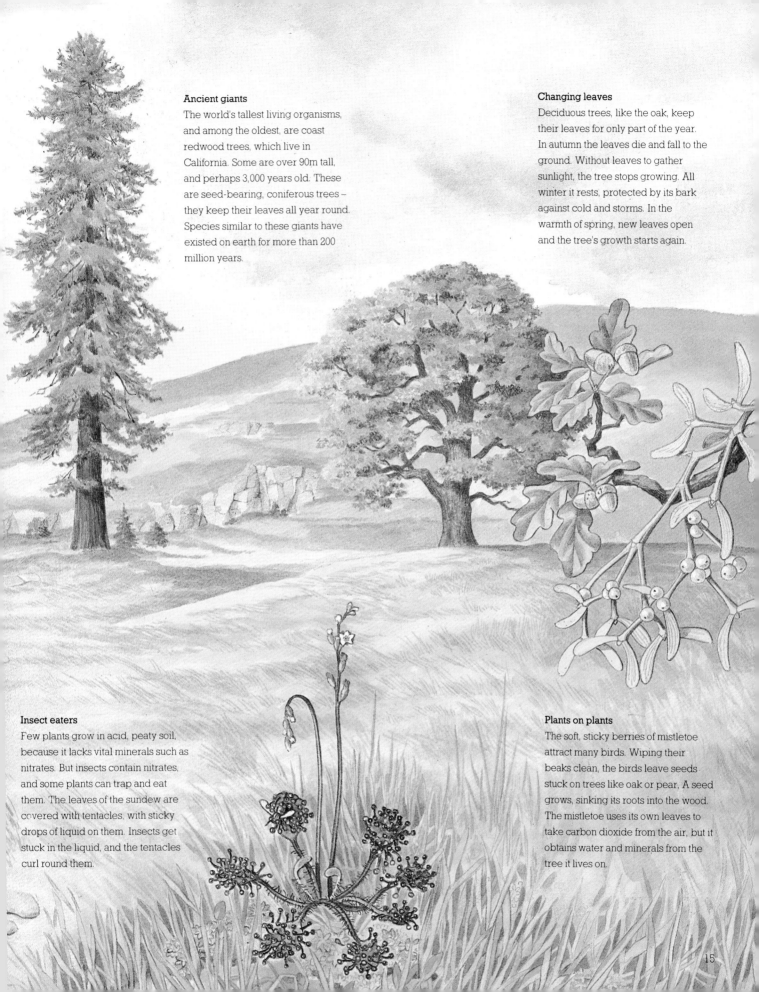

Ancient giants

The world's tallest living organisms, and among the oldest, are coast redwood trees, which live in California. Some are over 90m tall, and perhaps 3,000 years old. These are seed-bearing, coniferous trees – they keep their leaves all year round. Species similar to these giants have existed on earth for more than 200 million years.

Changing leaves

Deciduous trees, like the oak, keep their leaves for only part of the year. In autumn the leaves die and fall to the ground. Without leaves to gather sunlight, the tree stops growing. All winter it rests, protected by its bark against cold and storms. In the warmth of spring, new leaves open and the tree's growth starts again.

Insect eaters

Few plants grow in acid, peaty soil, because it lacks vital minerals such as nitrates. But insects contain nitrates, and some plants can trap and eat them. The leaves of the sundew are covered with tentacles, with sticky drops of liquid on them. Insects get stuck in the liquid, and the tentacles curl round them.

Plants on plants

The soft, sticky berries of mistletoe attract many birds. Wiping their beaks clean, the birds leave seeds stuck on trees like oak or pear. A seed grows, sinking its roots into the wood. The mistletoe uses its own leaves to take carbon dioxide from the air, but it obtains water and minerals from the tree it lives on.

15

Looking around

It is not just seeing with your eyes that tells you how the world looks. In your eyes, pictures made from waves of light are turned into electrical impulses, which pass along nerves to your brain. Your eyes alone make no sense of the pictures – in fact, because of the way they collect light waves, they see everything upside down and back to front. Your brain turns the pictures the right way round, and sorts out what they mean. Your eyes and brain work together to give you your vision of the world.

The world which you see is different from the world which any other creature sees. Different brains make sense of the world in different ways. You know what an insect looks like to you, but not what it looks like to a chameleon. It is food to the chameleon, that much is certain, but it is impossible to tell what else registers on the chameleon's brain.

The chameleon's scaled eyes swivel independently of each other. They can turn through 180 degrees, so it can see all round itself. They can focus sharply ahead of it. The chameleon moves slowly along a branch, protected by its camouflage, grasping with its feet. It sees an insect, and suddenly its long, sticky-tipped tongue flicks out and catches it. However weird the chameleon's eyes may look, they work with perfect precision. This combination of eyes and brain and tongue, and body highly adapted to life in trees, rarely misses its mark.

There are countless ways of seeing the world. The simplest eyes, like the light-sensitive cells on the skin of an earthworm, can see only the difference between light and dark. Dogs and horses see in shades of grey, bees can see ultra-violet light, which you cannot. Birds of prey see more detail than you, and many can see quite clearly when it is too dark for you to see at all. But always the eye leads inwards to the brain. It is the window between the outside world which all creatures share, and the inner view of it which is unique to each of us.

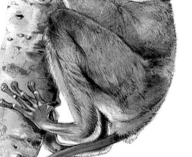

Tarsier
In the forests of south-east Asia, tarsiers come out at night looking for insects to eat. Their eyes are enormous, adapted to seeing in the dark. In comparison with the size of their heads, tarsiers have larger eyes than any other mammal. In fact, the area of the eye socket is greater than the area of the tarsier's stomach and brain combined.

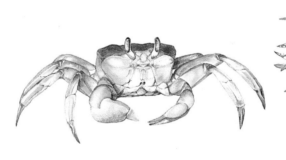
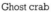

Ghost crab
Living at ground level in a world of swirling sand and sea-spray, ghost crabs come out of their burrows at low tide to feed between land and sea. In such a world, any delicate projection can easily be damaged, so the crabs have eyes on stalks which fold away safely into their shells, when they burrow or the sea breaks over them.

Squid
The eyes of a squid look almost human, though squids are molluscs, among the oldest forms of life on earth. A giant squid's eyes may measure 40cm across – larger than the largest dinner plate – and be able to see clearly at any distance. No other backboneless animal has such efficient eyes, which can make out finer details even than human eyes.

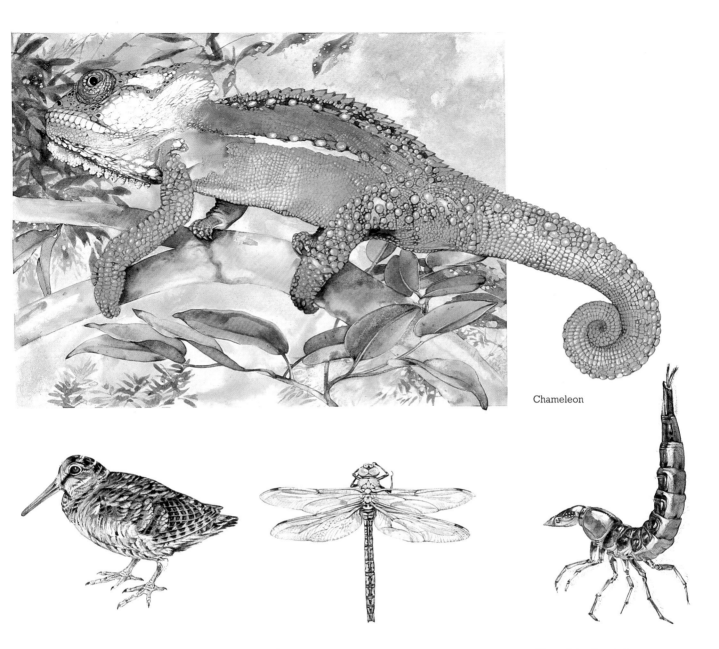

Chameleon

Woodcock

Its long, straight bill enables a woodcock to probe deep in the ground for worms. But in this position it is in great danger of being caught by predators. To give it all-round vision, when it is feeding or sitting on its nest, its bulging eyes are set towards the back of its head, so that it can see just as well backwards as forwards.

Dragonfly

The great, criss-cross patterned swellings covering most of a dragonfly's head are its eyes. These are not two single eyes, but more than 40,000 small, simple eyes. Each is a single cell, sensitive to light. All together they build up a mosaic picture of the world around the dragonfly, as it hunts down the insects on which it feeds.

Great diving beetle larva

The larva of a great diving beetle is a ferocious predator, killing and eating small fish, newts and other water insects with its tube-like jaws. It breathes and sees through its tail. Simple light-sensitive cells in its tail guide it back-end first to the surface to take in oxygen, and warn it of danger when the shadow of a bird falls on the water.

The world of sound

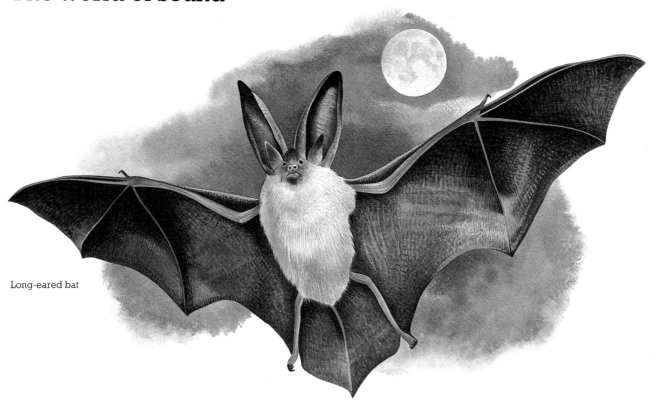

Long-eared bat

Most of what you know about the world, you find out with your eyes. Most of what a bat knows, it finds out with its ears. Close your eyes and listen, and you enter the world of the bat. You are very clumsy by comparison with the bat, stumbling in the dark. As a bat flies by night, it keeps up a stream of squeaks, too high for human ears to hear. It picks up echoes of the squeaks with its highly sensitive ears, mapping out the world around it. Just by listening to the echoes, it can flutter through the branches of a tree without ever hitting them, and catch moths and other insects to eat.

Though you cannot learn as much from sound as a bat, your ear is still a supremely delicate instrument for collecting information from the air. Every sound is a vibration, a wave travelling at some 1,200 km an hour in air, and four times faster in water. The wave enters your ear, gathered in by the flap on the outside. It reaches your eardrum – a tight membrane closing the channel into your head. The eardrum vibrates, moving three little bones, which knock on the inner ear. Here

a fluid moves in time to the knocking, activating nerve cells like tiny hairs. The cells set off electrical charges, which travel to your brain to be identified. Passing through your ear, the sound is made 22 times louder before the nerve cells translate it into the electrical language of your brain.

Sounds tell animals where there is food, where others of their species can be found, when there is a predator nearby. Fish hear with many tiny ears strung out along their bodies, dolphins use an echo-location system like that of bats. There are even some moths, with simple ears under their wings, which can hear the ultrasonic squeaks of bats. The moth dodges away from the sound of danger just as the bat closes in on the sound of food.

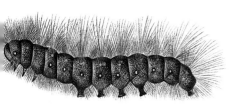

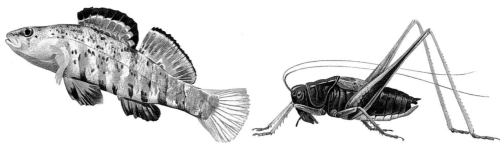

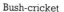

Woolly bear

Some caterpillars – including the woolly bear, caterpillar of the garden tiger moth – can detect sound waves with the sensitive hairs on their bodies, curling up tightly for safety. The hairs are also highly sensitive to touch, and make the caterpillar unpleasant for most birds and other predators to eat, like a mouthful of wriggling toothbrush.

Orangethroat darter

The lateral line along the side of a fish is like a row of miniature ears. Small openings along the line lead to a canal full of fluid in the fish's body. Here, sensory cells detect sound waves and other vibrations in the water around the fish, informing it about food and predators, and helping it to stay close to its shoal.

Bush-cricket

The chirruping noise made by a bush-cricket is a way of attracting a mate. The male rubs its wings together to make the sound, and the female hears it with ears on her forelegs. Small openings in the legs conduct the sound to the insect's central nervous system and brain. The female responds only to the mating call of males of her own species.

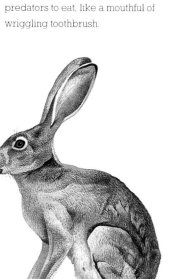

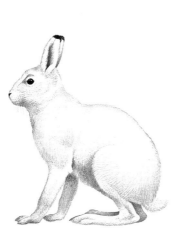

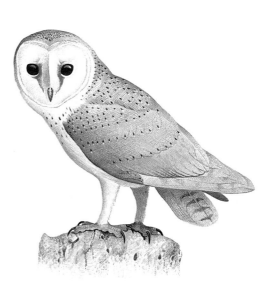

Jack rabbit

All hares rely on their acute hearing and sense of smell to warn them of danger. But American jack rabbits – really hares, in spite of the name – have another use for their enormous ears. They live in the desert, and their sparsely furred ears, with a network of blood vessels, help to keep them cool by continuously losing unwanted body heat.

Arctic hare

In contrast with jack rabbits, Arctic hares must conserve as much body heat as they can, if they are to survive the freezing, ice-locked winters of their northern homeland. So their ears are small, and warmly wrapped in fur. What the hares lose in hearing, they make up with camouflage, turning snow-white in winter as a protection against predators.

Barn owl

Flying on almost silent wings through the still night, barn owls hunt their prey more by ear than by any other sense. Even in complete darkness they can pinpoint and catch mice just by listening. The ears are openings in the sides of the owl's head, without earflaps, and one is higher than the other, to help the owl judge distances accurately.

Chemical pictures

The world is always full of smells, which make invisible pictures around you of what is happening now, and what happened just before. The pictures are millions of floating chemical particles, which you trap with your nose. In the roof of your nose the particles are caught on nerve endings like little brushes, and dissolved in fluid. The nerves pass messages to your brain, which identifies the smell. You can distinguish between hundreds, perhaps thousands, of smells. Even so, you cannot smell as much as many other creatures. A dog standing beside you, straining its head forwards and sniffing intensely, can smell vivid pictures of the world which you are not aware of at all. Some moths can detect the scent of their mates from as much as 8km away.

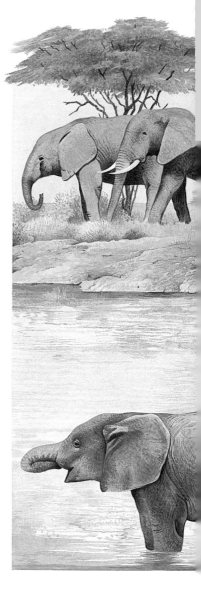

An elephant, holding its trunk in the air, receives wind-borne scents from far away, smelling into the distance. By sweeping its trunk over the ground, it can smell what is happening there. No other nose quite compares with an elephant's trunk. Not only is it acutely sensitive to smell, but it also serves as a hand, a jug, a shower and a trumpet. It is made of thousands of muscles, more than you have in your whole body. It is immensely strong, yet capable of the greatest delicacy and gentleness.

Taste and smell are very alike – sometimes it is hard to tell the difference between them. When you have a cold, and your nose is blocked, you can hardly taste what you eat, because you can hardly smell it. Taste, like smell, is a chemical sense. On your tongue you dissolve chemicals, to find out if they are sweet or sour, salt or bitter. In your nose you dissolve them, to smell if they are flowery or fruity, spicy, smoky or just plain bad.

Indian cobra

Snakes have nostrils and can smell in the ordinary way. They can also smell by flicking their tongues in and out, gathering chemical particles from the air. These are passed from the tongue to special pits in the snake's mouth. Impulses are then sent to the snake's brain, which identifies the scent in the air.

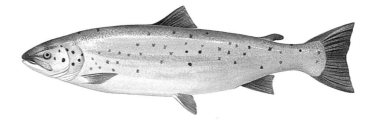

Atlantic salmon

For the first part of its life an Atlantic salmon lives in the river where it was born. Then it migrates to the sea, and spends several years there. Finally it returns across the ocean to breed in the same river, guided back by the long-remembered smell of the river water, spreading through the ocean.

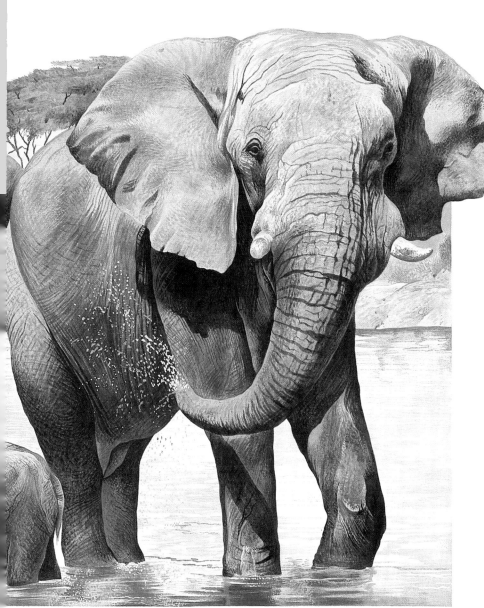

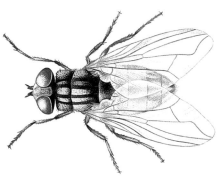

Elephant

House-fly

For a house-fly there is really no difference between smelling and tasting – it does both, in one, with its feet. When it lands on food, chemical receptors on the soles of its feet tell it what the food is like. If the taste and smell are right, the fly's tongue flicks out and it automatically starts feeding.

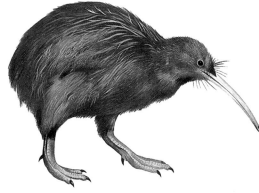

Kiwi

Most birds have a poor sense of smell. But the flightless kiwi is different. At night it wanders round the forests of New Zealand, probing the earth and fallen leaves with its long beak. At the tip of the beak is its nose – perfectly positioned for sniffing out worms, insects or fruit on the forest floor.

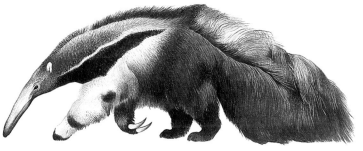

Anteater

Ants have a distinctive smell – this is one way in which they communicate. It also enables anteaters to track them down. Trotting along with its nose near the ground, an anteater is alert for the smell of food. When the smell comes, the anteater digs furiously, then licks up the ants with its long, snake-like tongue.

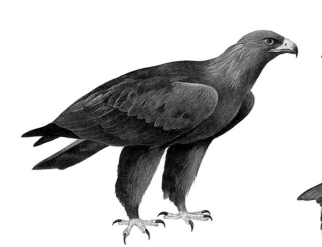

All beak and eyes

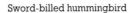

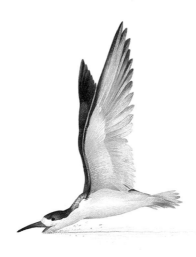

Golden eagle

The powerful, thick beak of a golden eagle, with a sharp, downward-pointing hook at the tip, is designed for gripping and tearing meat. The bird kills with its claws, pouncing on rabbits, hares, grouse and other birds. Perched on the dead body, it rips muscle and sinew off the bone.

Sword-billed hummingbird

Hovering in front of the long, bright trumpet of a tropical flower, the sword-billed hummingbird dips its beak deep inside, feeding on the flower's nectar. Compared with its body it has the longest beak in the world – its body is less than 8cm long, its beak is over 12cm.

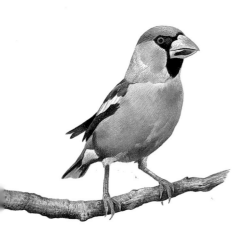

Hawfinch

The soft, tasty seeds of many plants are hidden in hard, protective shells – but with its highly developed face muscles and immense, nut-cracker beak, a hawfinch can crush stones as tough as an olive's or a cherry's. Almost all finches are seed-eaters, with beaks adapted for opening particular kinds of seed.

Skimmer

The most peculiar thing about a skimmer's beak is that the lower part is much larger than the upper part, making it unique among all birds' beaks. The gull-like bird dives down and skims just above the surface of a river, ploughing the lower part of its beak through the water and scooping up small fish.

Birds are the only animals on earth with feathers, but the earliest fossil animal known to have had feathers was unlike any bird living today. Archaeopteryx lived 140 million years ago, and it was half like a bird and half like a reptile. It had claws on its wings, scales on its head, and jaws full of teeth. In the course of evolution, birds' faces and bodies have assumed all kinds of forms – but not one has teeth. The nearest a bird comes to having teeth is when it is still inside the egg. A hard lump grows at the tip of its beak, which it uses to break out of the shell. Within days this egg-tooth disappears.

Beaks are adapted for eating, and one of the oddest of them all is the flamingo's. Though it looks clumsy, this beak makes it possible for flamingoes to feed in water full of chemicals, which would poison most birds. Water is sucked into the beak, then pumped out again. Food is trapped on bristle filters inside it. Frequently flamingoes rinse out their beaks in fresh water.

All birds' faces, like the flamingo's, are nearly all beak and eyes. Birds must see well in order to fly, and they live such active lives that they must eat nearly all the time. But they use their beaks for more than just eating. A beak can be a hand for carrying, a weapon for attack and defence, a tool for nest-building, a comb for looking after feathers, and even a showy ornament for attracting a mate.

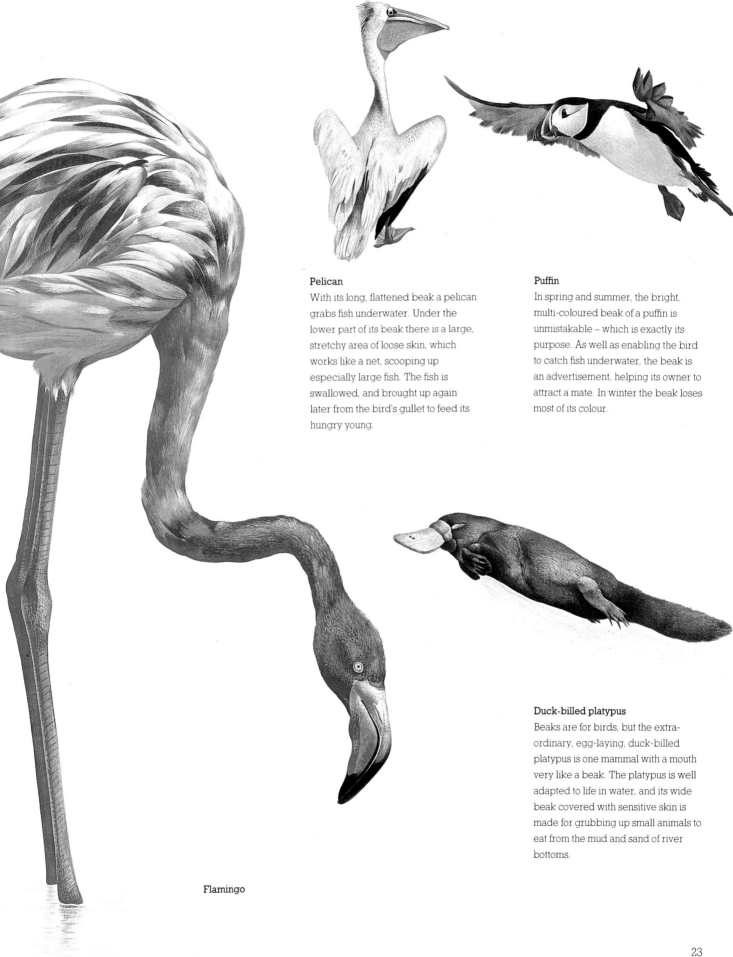

Pelican

With its long, flattened beak a pelican grabs fish underwater. Under the lower part of its beak there is a large, stretchy area of loose skin, which works like a net, scooping up especially large fish. The fish is swallowed, and brought up again later from the bird's gullet to feed its hungry young.

Puffin

In spring and summer, the bright, multi-coloured beak of a puffin is unmistakable – which is exactly its purpose. As well as enabling the bird to catch fish underwater, the beak is an advertisement, helping its owner to attract a mate. In winter the beak loses most of its colour.

Duck-billed platypus

Beaks are for birds, but the extra-ordinary, egg-laying, duck-billed platypus is one mammal with a mouth very like a beak. The platypus is well adapted to life in water, and its wide beak covered with sensitive skin is made for grubbing up small animals to eat from the mud and sand of river bottoms.

Flamingo

Open wide

Viper

Two enormous teeth in a viper's top jaw shoot poison into its prey. They are over 2.5cm long, and lie flat when the viper's mouth is closed. A bone swings them into position when the viper opens its mouth. The teeth are hollow. At the moment of impact, poison is injected into the victim's flesh.

Sea-urchin

Bristling spines and a hard shell protect sea-urchins from danger. Under the shell is the sea-urchin's mouth, with five protruding white teeth, immensely strong and reinforced with iron-salt. Sea-urchins' teeth, mouths and muscles have such power that they can bite algae from rocks and grind them up to eat.

Tiger

The canines – the dagger-shaped teeth on either side of the sharp, front incisors – are highly developed in meat-eaters such as tigers. The teeth are used for gripping, killing and ripping prey. Tigers swallow meat without chewing it, using their sharp back teeth as well as the front ones to tear and cut it.

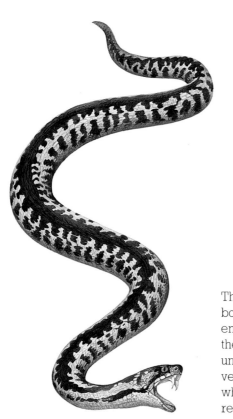
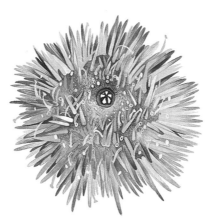
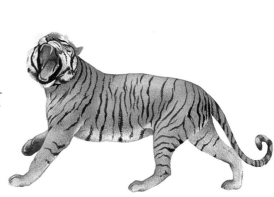

The hardest part of your body, harder than bone, almost as hard as glass, is the white enamel on the surface of your teeth. Under the enamel there is ivory-like toothbone; under that there is a soft area with blood vessels and nerves. You grow 20 milk teeth when you are a baby, which are later replaced by 32 permanent teeth. With your sharp front teeth, called incisors, you cut your food. With your dagger-shaped canines you tear it. With your bumpy back molars you chew it. You use your teeth for speaking clearly as well as for eating – the letters s, f, v and t are hard to say without teeth. Your teeth stop growing when they reach a certain size, and once lost they can never be replaced. But the front teeth of some mammals which feed on plants keep growing all their lives, being worn down by constant chewing.

A shark's teeth are different. A great white shark has row upon row of serrated, triangular, arrowhead teeth, which keep growing all the time. They move forwards in the shark's mouth as they grow, falling out when they lose their sharpness, being replaced by new teeth from behind. In its lifetime a shark uses up thousands of teeth. Most of its teeth lie flat until it bites into its prey. Then a membrane pulls them up into the ripping position. Because of the way the teeth slope backwards, a shark can never let go of what it bites until the flesh is torn apart.

Sharks were probably among the first animals on earth to have teeth, for teeth are thought to have evolved from fish's scales. Even on its skin a shark has hooked, sharp scales like teeth, as if its mouth were open all over its body.

Coypu

If a coypu or any other rodent stopped gnawing, its front teeth would grow so long that the lower ones would grow up into its head, and kill it. Coypus feed on plants, gnawing and chewing constantly. Like all rodents, they chew by moving their teeth backwards and forwards, not up and down as you do.

Babirusa

No one knows why the babirusa has such enormous, curved canine teeth, but they are certainly no use for eating or as weapons, because they curve dangerously back at its skull. The upper canines grow upwards in its mouth, breaking through the flesh and skin just below its eyes.

Walrus

The upper canines of a male walrus grow up to a metre long. The walrus uses them to keep marauding polar bears at bay, to keep open breathing holes in the Arctic ice, and to rake the sea-bed for shellfish to eat. It also uses them to help haul its huge body, which weighs about a tonne, out of the sea on to rock or ice.

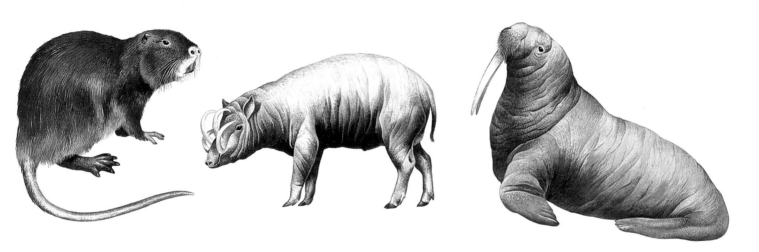

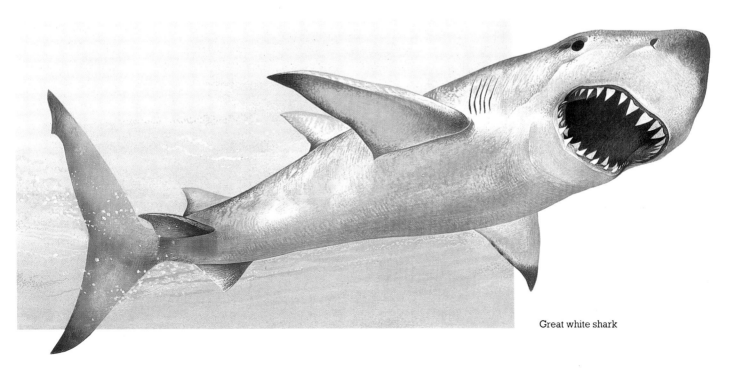

Great white shark

Dressed in horns

Animals attack with their teeth or claws, they stab, poison, trap, lure, suffocate, crush, suck blood, eat alive or even, among some fish, generate electrical shocks to kill their prey. In defence they are no less inventive, running, hiding, burrowing, leaping, pretending to be rocks, sticks, leaves or dewdrops, or looking fiercer or more poisonous than they really are. They live in constant danger of being eaten, and in constant need to eat. They are all, in some way, armed to survive.

Having horns is like carrying a dangerous weapon for everyone to see. Often this is pure bluff. The male Hercules beetle can grow more than 15cm long, making it one of the largest beetles in the world. Almost half of its length is accounted for by its horns. They seem to be little real use in attack or defence. Sometimes males use them like rather clumsy forceps to carry off the much smaller females, but beetle courtship happens just as successfully without such displays of brute force. In the end the horns seem to be no more than an extravagant male boast, a sort of loud, beetle way of dressing up to look strong, or of attracting females.

There are many other creatures with appendages which look like horns, but which serve very different purposes. The antennae of insects are mainly used to detect smells in the air. The horns of a snail are really eyes on stalks, and the horn of an angler fish is a lure to attract its prey.

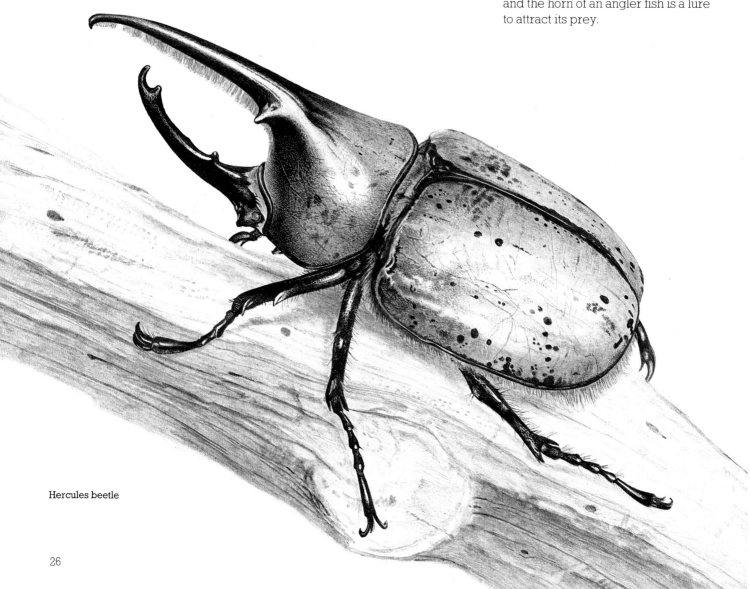

Hercules beetle

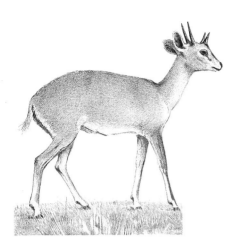

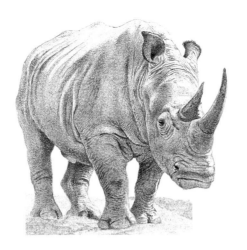

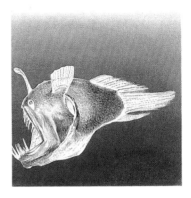

Four-horned antelope

The only mammal in the world with four horns is the chousingha, or four-horned antelope, from India. Two of its horns are in the normal place, by its ears, but the other two are between its eyes. The horns keep growing throughout the animal's life – but why there are four of them remains uncertain.

Rhinoceros

The horn of a rhinoceros is not made of horn, or bone, at all. It develops from a tight bundle of fibres – the same material that makes feathers – growing like hairs from the skin above the rhino's nose. For the sake of their horns, believed to make a powerful love potion, rhinos have been hunted almost to extinction.

Angler fish

What looks like a horn above the angler fish's upper lip is really part of a fin, turned into a fishing rod. Even the wriggling bait on the rod is part of the fish's body. When another fish swims close, to investigate the lure, the angler fish swallows violently, sucking in water and prey alike.

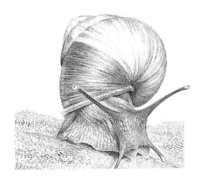

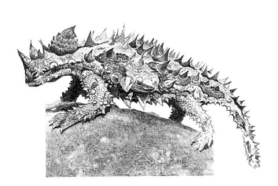

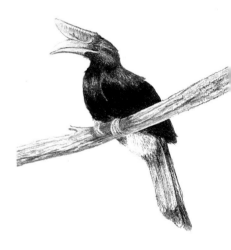

Snail

When a snail comes out of its shell, four horns unfurl on its head. The upper ones are simple eyes on stalks, the lower ones are to help it feel its way. Probably the snail can see little more with its periscope eyes than the difference between light and dark, and perhaps the haziest flickering of movement.

Thorny devil

Spiked horns bristle all over the skin of the Australian thorny devil, making it a mouthful which few predators would ever take. The lizard eats ants, and uses its armour only in self-defence. If attacked, it stands still and tucks its head between its forelegs, lifting the lump on its neck to face its attacker.

Rhinoceros hornbill

Clattering through the high treetops of an Asian tropical forest, it seems a wonder that the rhinoceros hornbill can fly at all, with such a bill and such a horn on top of it. In fact the horn is almost hollow, and reinforced with struts, so it weighs hardly anything. Its only use is as an ornament for display.

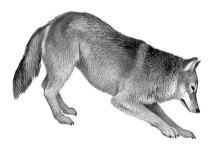

Wolf

In a single night wolves may run as far as 60 km, following or searching for their prey. Their claws are exposed to constant wear and tear, but they catch the ground as the wolf runs, providing grip like a runner's spiked shoes. And when the wolf leaps to kill, biting for its victim's throat, its claws give it extra power.

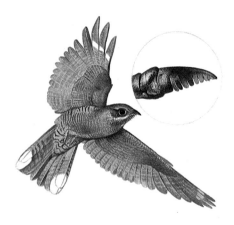

Nightjar

On the end of its middle toe a nightjar has a serrated, comb-like claw. It uses this while grooming its feathers, to keep them free of dust, and also to keep clean and untangled the special bristles which grow around its mouth. As it flies along with its mouth wide open, these bristles help it to catch insects.

Hanging around

Your nails are made of keratin, a substance also found in animals' horns and birds' feathers. They grow from living roots, hidden under the skin, at the rate of about 2cm a year. Except for their roots, the nails are dead – built up of layers of closely-packed, dead cells. They protect the sensitive ends of your fingers and toes, and have other simple functions like picking or scratching. But they are nothing compared with the great, hooked claws of the three-toed sloth, without which the sloth could not live at all.

Even when a sloth is asleep – and it sleeps some 18 hours a day, hanging upside down in trees – its claws clamp it so securely to the tree that hardly anything can dislodge it. Sloths do everything

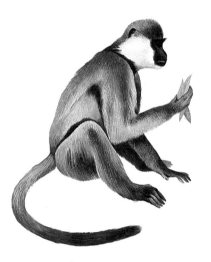

Capped langur

The fingers and toes of all monkeys and apes – including human beings, who are descended from ape-like ancestors – have very sensitive tips, protected by nails. The capped langur from south-east Asia is no exception – it has nails not very different from yours. It eats leaves and lives almost entirely in trees.

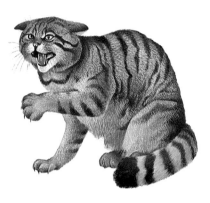

Wild cat

Lashing out with its paws, a wild cat can inflict terrible damage with its needle-sharp claws; but as it pads across the ground, it can draw them back into special sheaths. When it climbs trees, hunting for birds to eat, its claws give it a secure footing, and a firm grip once the bird has been caught.

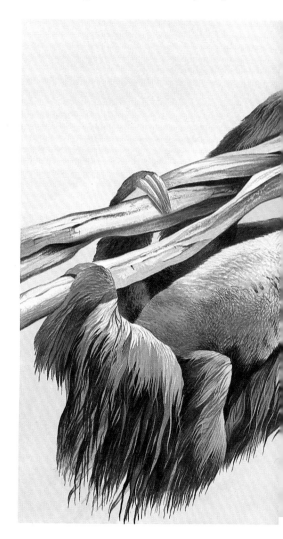

slowly, and live almost entirely upside down. They eat, mate, give birth and walk long bony limb after long bony limb – all slowly, all upside down, hooked on by their claws. They eat leaves and live alone, and their fur grows in the opposite direction to the fur of other animals, so that the water just runs off them when it rains. They are not easily provoked – hearing little, seeing little, apparently feeling little. Their stillness hides them from predators' eyes, and moths and algae growing in their fur complete the camouflage. But if danger does come near, or even if one sloth invades the sleepy privacy of another, one swing of a long bent arm turns the claws from animal coathangers into deadly cutting blades.

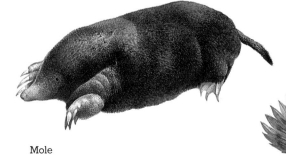

Mole

Its spade-like hands, short, strong arms and tough, scooping claws give the mole its unique ability as a burrower. It lives almost entirely underground, and can shovel through more than 15 metres of earth in less than an hour. Just the faint vibration of a worm moving in the earth can start it drilling hungrily forwards.

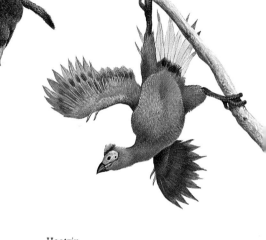

Hoatzin

A young hoatzin has claws on its wings, like Archaeopteryx, the first feathered animal known to have lived on earth. It uses these wing-claws to help it clamber about in trees and bushes, and to leave and return to its nest before it can fly. But the claws do not stay with it for long, disappearing after a few weeks.

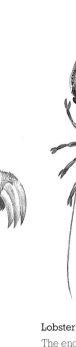

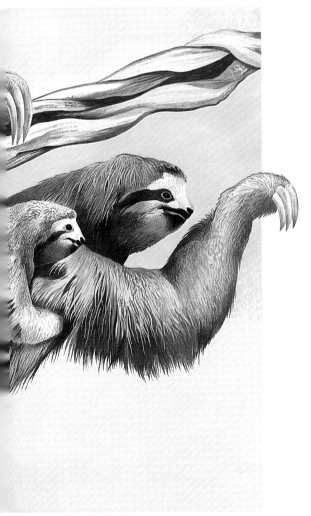

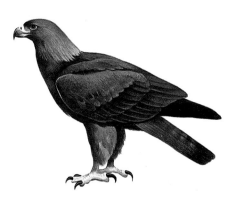

Lobster

The enormous claws, or pincers, of a lobster are used for grabbing and crushing prey, or for picking meat off dead bodies. Often one claw is larger than the other. The large claw is for smashing, the smaller one is for picking and grabbing. If a lobster loses a claw, a new one can grow to replace it.

Golden eagle

When a flying eagle spots its prey – perhaps a hare running across moorland, or a grouse breaking from heather – it drops swiftly, and dives in with its talons outstretched. Its hooked claws are razor sharp. When the bird hits its quarry, the claws close in a killing grip from which no animal ever escapes.

Three-toed sloth

Down on the ground

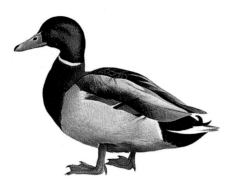

Mallard

Wide webs between the toes of waterfowl turn their feet into flippers for swimming. The mallard's body is also well adapted for swimming – its long, torpedo shape slides smoothly through the water. But on land the set and balance of the duck's body is awkward and top-heavy, and its feet are clumsy, like shoes which are many sizes too large.

When you walk, first you hit the ground with one heel. You pass the weight of your body down the outside edge of your foot, then shift it across the front to your big toe. You push with your toe just as the other heel hits the ground. Your feet are one of the boniest parts of your body – between them they have 52 bones, about a quarter of your skeleton. On these bones you walk, run, hop and jump, you dance and play football, you can keep standing upright as long as you can stay awake. They work so easily with your muscles, and put such spring and precision into your stride, that moving across the ground is as smooth as if you had tyres.

Millions of years ago your ancestors were probably living in trees. When they first came down to live on the ground, it is possible that they used their hands as well as their feet for walking, as other apes do today. Some time they took to walking upright, which set their hands free to do other things, like making tools, or carrying food from place to place. If they lived on the plains, they would also be able to see further by standing upright – to spot both predators and prey. Fossil footprints found in Tanzania show that man-like animals were walking upright more than three million years ago. The print of the big toe is unmistakable, pushing the body forwards with every stride, pushing the animal forwards to becoming a human being.

When a flying frog comes down from the trees the story is very different. Between its toes there are wide webs, which it spreads out as it leaps. It glides on its feet through the air, planing from one tree to another, perhaps as far as 15 metres away. This is one special way the frog has of moving, and of escaping when danger threatens. Its feet become little, fixed wings, as yours become turning wheels.

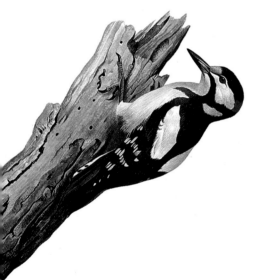

Great spotted woodpecker

Most birds have three toes pointing forwards and one backwards, which gives them a strong grip in trees and steady balance on the ground. In order to cling to tree trunks and to climb vertically, woodpeckers have two toes in front and two behind.

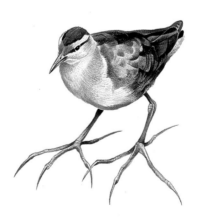

Lily trotter

A lily pad floating on the water could never support a lily trotter's weight, if the bird did not have such long toes. But the toes spread its weight out evenly, and it uses the lily pads as stepping stones as it searches for insects to eat.

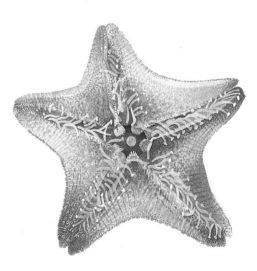

Starfish

Each of a starfish's arms is covered underneath with hundreds of feet – little tubes which are worked by water pressure. The tubes hold on by suction, extending and retracting to move the starfish forwards, at a top speed of some 15cm a minute.

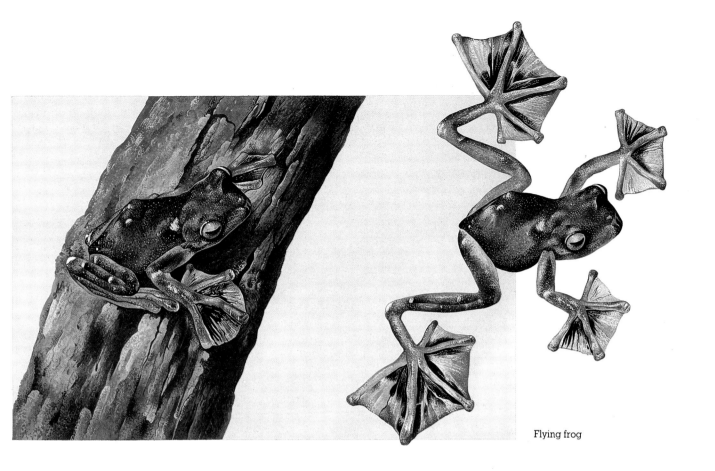

Flying frog

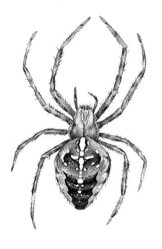
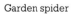

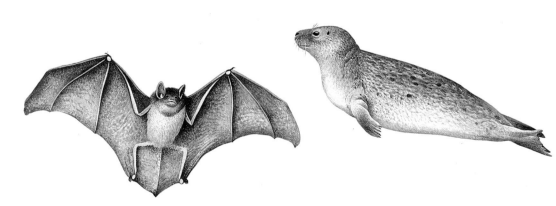

Garden spider

When an insect flies into a garden spider's web, it is the glue on most of the threads which catches it. The spider's feet are such a delicate arrangement of claws and bristles that it can run across the web treading only on the few dry threads.

Disc-winged bat

On its feet, and on the front of its wings, a disc-winged bat has large suckers, which enable it to hang securely upside down, even when it is asleep. The suckers are so strong that just one of them is enough to support the bat's full weight.

Grey seal

In the water a seal moves with ease, grace and power, but on land its body becomes slow and ungainly. Its legs and feet are little use for walking. They are partly enclosed in its body, partly flattened, webbed between the toes and wrapped in thick, rubbery skin.

Different endings

The smell of a male ring-tailed lemur goes ahead of it into battle. When males fight, first they smear their tails with scent secreted from glands in their wrists and armpits. Then they face one another, waving their tails in the air and fanning their smell forwards. In fact they may not come to grips with one another at all, but just let the stink do all the fighting.

A tail can be a stinking flag, like the lemur's, or an extra limb for holding on to branches, or a seat to sit on, or a glorious ornament, or a device to help with balance or steering; or it can be, as yours is, something which vanished during the course of evolution, millions of years ago. In general ground-living monkeys have less use for their tails than monkeys which live in trees, and many do not have tails at all. Human beings and monkeys evolved from a common ancestor, which probably had a tail. But if a tail, or any part of the body, is no longer useful, the processes of evolution usually get rid of it.

But it is not quite true that you never have a tail. When you are still in your mother's womb you have a tail, which is quite long at first, and only disappears some time in the fourth month. The tail is an echo from millions of years ago, a ghostly reminder of the past. But now, and all your life, all that remains of it is your coccyx – the little, pointed bone where your back ends.

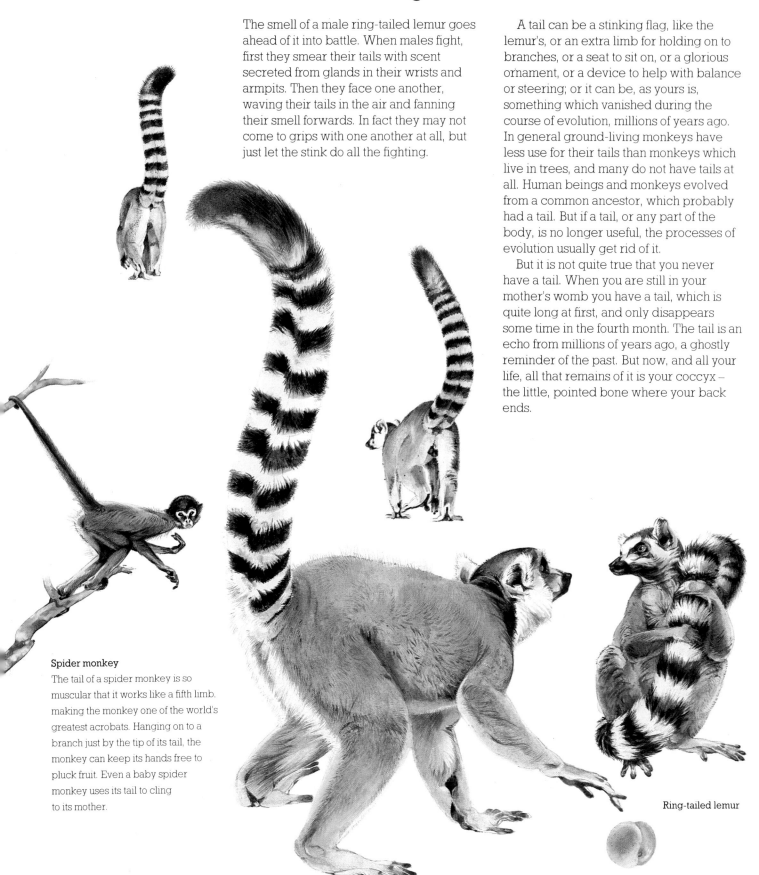

Spider monkey
The tail of a spider monkey is so muscular that it works like a fifth limb, making the monkey one of the world's greatest acrobats. Hanging on to a branch just by the tip of its tail, the monkey can keep its hands free to pluck fruit. Even a baby spider monkey uses its tail to cling to its mother.

Ring-tailed lemur

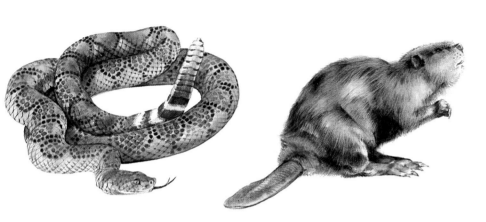
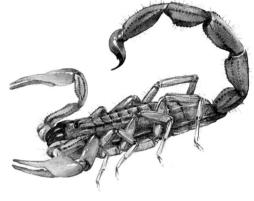

Rattlesnake

No one chooses to disturb a rattlesnake, nor does the snake wish to be disturbed. By rattling the pieces of hollow, dry skin at the end of its tail, it gives warning of its presence, reserving the poison in its fangs for its prey. The rattle is a message of peace from one of the deadliest snakes of all.

Beaver

If a beaver sees danger approaching – perhaps a hungry bear or a pack of wolves – it takes to the water and dives out of sight, first slapping its wide, scaly tail on the water to warn its neighbours. The tail works as a rudder, and on land it props up and balances the beaver as it cuts down trees to build dams.

Scorpion

At night scorpions come out from their daytime hiding places to hunt their prey – insects, spiders and sometimes other scorpions; or else they lurk, waiting, in their lairs. They grab the prey with their pincers, then whip their long tails forward over their backs, delivering a sting which kills or paralyses.

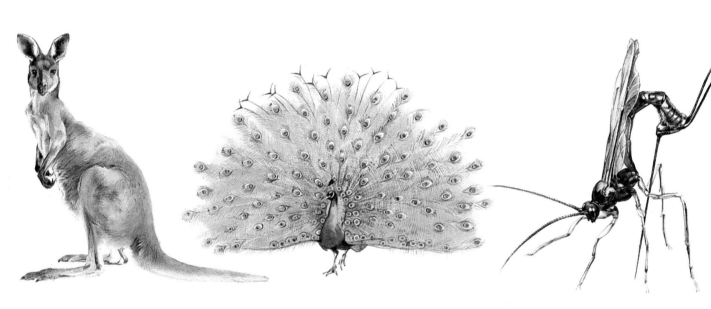

Kangaroo

As a kangaroo bounds across the Australian bush, covering more than 6m with every leap and reaching speeds of up to 60kph, it leans well forwards and balances itself with its long, heavy tail. When it comes to a halt, it can lean back on its tail, which is strong enough to support its weight.

Peacock

The brilliant green and blue tail feathers of a peacock, twinkling with iridescent eyespots, are a fan to attract a female. Usually the feathers are kept folded, trailing along the ground. But in the mating season the male raises and spreads them, shaking its wings in order to make the colours shimmer.

Ichneumon wasp

When a female ichneumon wasp is ready to lay her eggs, she seeks out the place in a tree where a beetle grub is hidden. With the long, thin, sharp tube at the end of her body, she drills into the wood, and lays her egg next to the grub, or even inside it. When the egg hatches, the wasp larva eats the beetle.

Between two worlds

A plover lands beside a Nile crocodile, basking open-mouthed in the sunshine. The bird walks about the crocodile, feeding on flies which the crocodile has disturbed. It may even pick food from between the crocodile's teeth. The bird must eat, as often as it can – the pace of its life, and the way its body works, make it almost continuously hungry. The crocodile must eat too, but not nearly so often. It needs sunshine much more than food. So the plover is really quite safe so close to the crocodile's mouth.

The plover is covered with feathers, the crocodile with scales, and there is more to this difference than meets the eye. The inner temperature of a bird's body is always the same, maintained by complicated systems inside it. Its feathers insulate it from the outside world, keeping it warm in cold weather and cool when it is hot. A crocodile, by contrast, has no fixed temperature. The sun beating on its scales warms it up, inside as well as out. If it gets too hot, it goes into the water. Having its mouth open helps to cool it. At night it lies in the warm river. Its scales collect heat from outside, as the plover's feathers conserve heat which is already there.

You are warm-blooded, like the plover or the impalas in the distance, and most of what you eat feeds the systems which keep your temperature constant at 37°C. Your skin is a barrier between two worlds – the regulated world inside you, and the fluctuating world outside. When you shiver or sweat, you are looking after the inner world, warming it or cooling it. When you come out in goose pimples, you are activating the same muscles that a furry

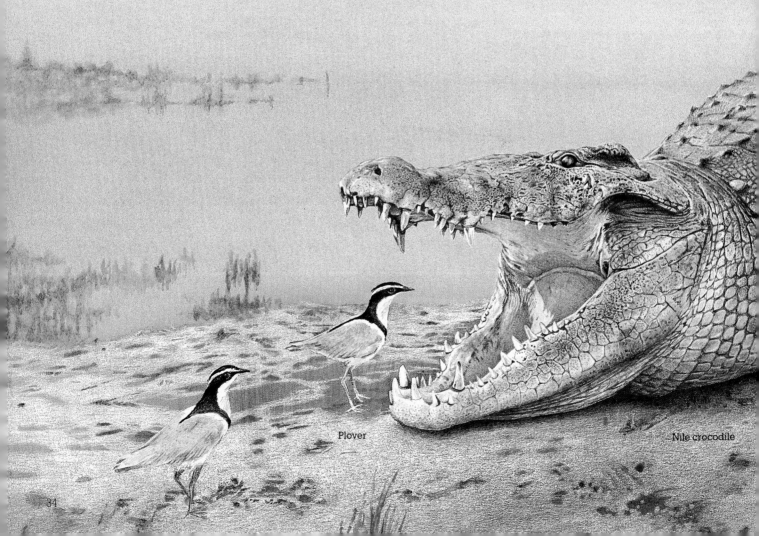

Plover

Nile crocodile

animal uses to make its hairs stand out in the cold, or a bird uses to fluff up its feathers. These, too, are ways of keeping warm.

But your skin is not just for keeping your temperature constant. It keeps body fluids in, and water out. It protects you from injury, bacteria and the ultra-violet rays of the sun. It is full of nerves, and never stops informing your brain about heat, cold, pressure, pain and touch. In these ways it perceives the world. Hair and nails grow from it, providing more protection. Sweat and special oils spring from it. It is thinnest over your eyelids – about 0.5mm thick. On the soles of your feet it may be as much as 6mm thick. Wherever it is, the outer layer

is made up of dead cells, which flake off continuously, floating away as dust in the air. They are replaced by other cells, also dead, from below. In less than a month your outside changes completely.

You are naked, now and for ever. But your skin looks after you like a friend, as some sort of outer covering looks after every living thing on earth – as bark looks after a tree, as an external skeleton looks after an insect, as skin and fur look after an impala, as skin and feathers look after a plover, as scales feed a crocodile on sunshine.

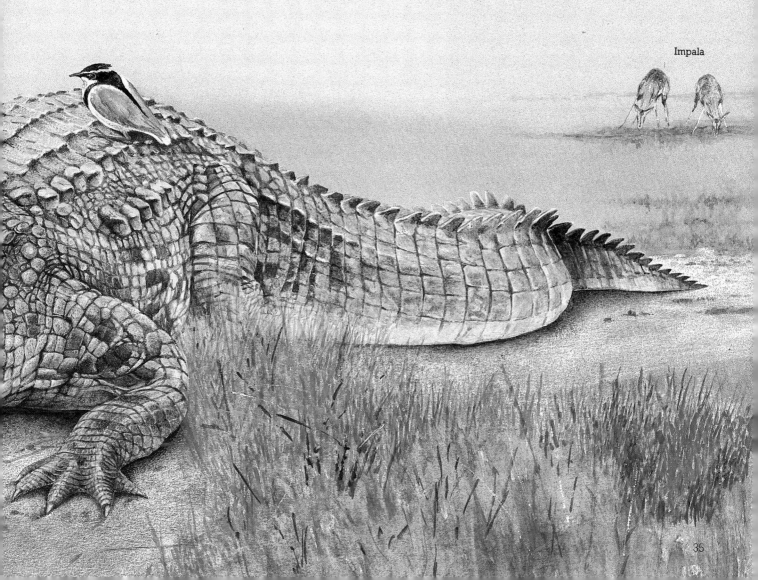

Impala

The light in your eyes

White light is everywhere, made of all the colours of the rainbow. Light strikes something, and is reflected into your eyes. You see a colour. Different wavelengths of light make different colours. When raindrops split up the wavelengths, a rainbow appears. When all the wavelengths are absorbed by something, you see black. When you look at a field of grass and see green, this is because grass reflects the green wavelengths. It uses the other colours, particularly red and blue, in the process of making food. Grass is green because it has no use for green light.

Every colour tells a story in nature. The brilliant blue of a kingfisher is a reminder to predators that its flesh tastes foul. The black and yellow of a wasp is a reminder that wasps sting. A hoverfly has no sting, but it looks like a wasp. By evolving its colours, it has gained protection from the wasp. Many birds will avoid it, for fear of the sting which it looks as if it has.

A trout is dappled brown so that it is hard for a predator to see against the riverbed. Frogs, too, are often coloured to merge with their surroundings. On the plains of Africa, a distant herd of zebras achieves another effect – looking like a mass of stripes, not animals at all, half lost in a shimmering heat haze. These animals use colour to hide themselves, as others use it to make sure that they are seen, because they are dangerous, or taste unpleasant, or want to attract a mate.

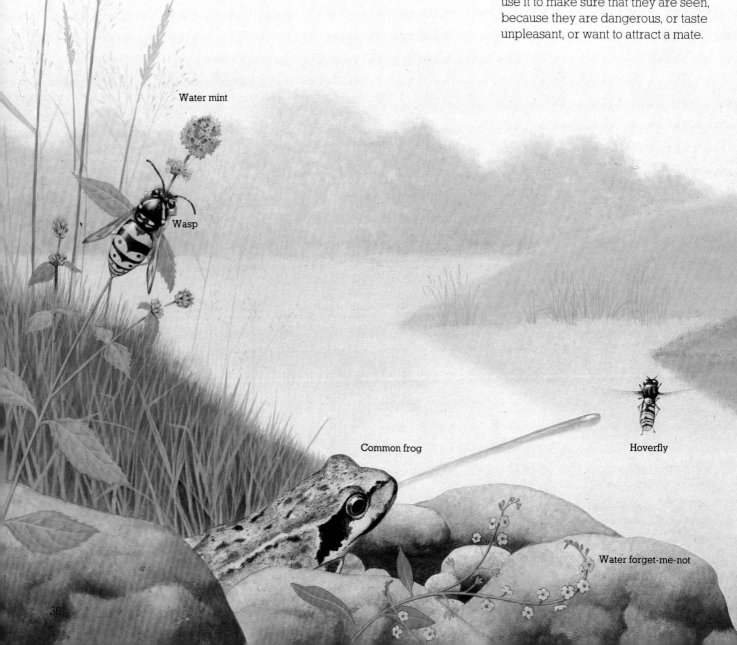

Water mint

Wasp

Common frog

Hoverfly

Water forget-me-not

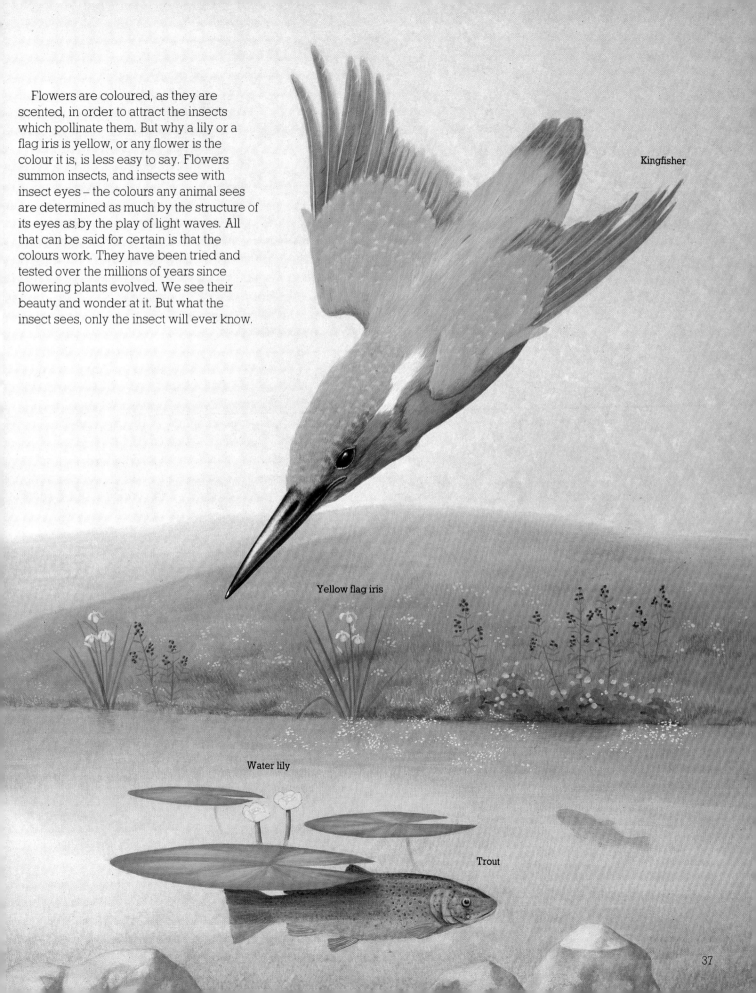

Flowers are coloured, as they are scented, in order to attract the insects which pollinate them. But why a lily or a flag iris is yellow, or any flower is the colour it is, is less easy to say. Flowers summon insects, and insects see with insect eyes – the colours any animal sees are determined as much by the structure of its eyes as by the play of light waves. All that can be said for certain is that the colours work. They have been tried and tested over the millions of years since flowering plants evolved. We see their beauty and wonder at it. But what the insect sees, only the insect will ever know.

Kingfisher

Yellow flag iris

Water lily

Trout

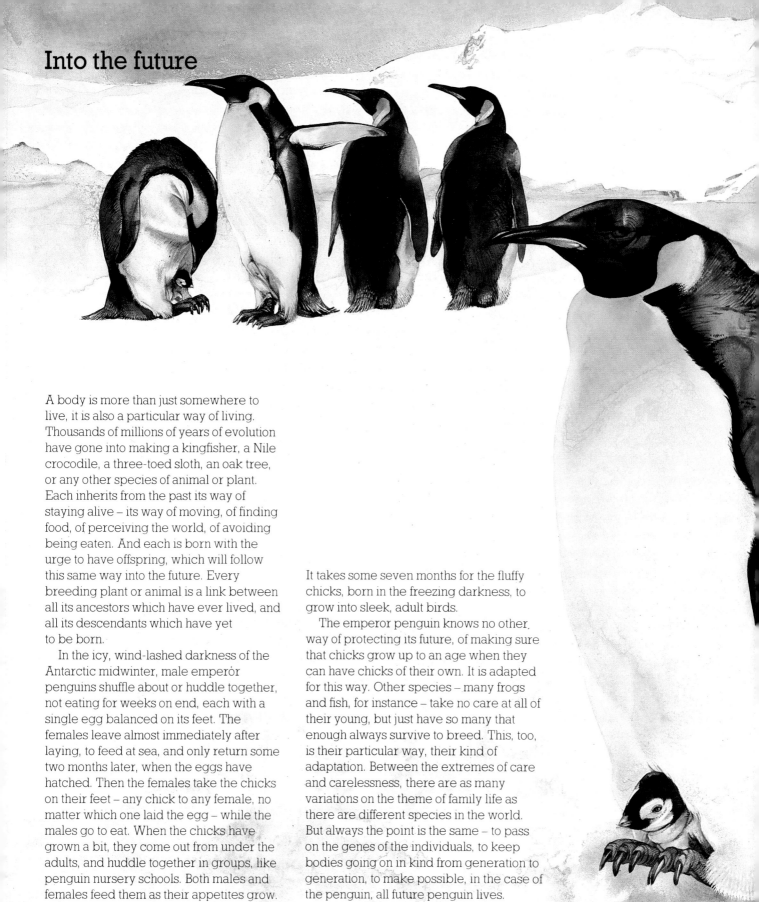

Into the future

A body is more than just somewhere to live, it is also a particular way of living. Thousands of millions of years of evolution have gone into making a kingfisher, a Nile crocodile, a three-toed sloth, an oak tree, or any other species of animal or plant. Each inherits from the past its way of staying alive – its way of moving, of finding food, of perceiving the world, of avoiding being eaten. And each is born with the urge to have offspring, which will follow this same way into the future. Every breeding plant or animal is a link between all its ancestors which have ever lived, and all its descendants which have yet to be born.

In the icy, wind-lashed darkness of the Antarctic midwinter, male emperor penguins shuffle about or huddle together, not eating for weeks on end, each with a single egg balanced on its feet. The females leave almost immediately after laying, to feed at sea, and only return some two months later, when the eggs have hatched. Then the females take the chicks on their feet – any chick to any female, no matter which one laid the egg – while the males go to eat. When the chicks have grown a bit, they come out from under the adults, and huddle together in groups, like penguin nursery schools. Both males and females feed them as their appetites grow.

It takes some seven months for the fluffy chicks, born in the freezing darkness, to grow into sleek, adult birds.

The emperor penguin knows no other way of protecting its future, of making sure that chicks grow up to an age when they can have chicks of their own. It is adapted for this way. Other species – many frogs and fish, for instance – take no care at all of their young, but just have so many that enough always survive to breed. This, too, is their particular way, their kind of adaptation. Between the extremes of care and carelessness, there are as many variations on the theme of family life as there are different species in the world. But always the point is the same – to pass on the genes of the individuals, to keep bodies going on in kind from generation to generation, to make possible, in the case of the penguin, all future penguin lives.

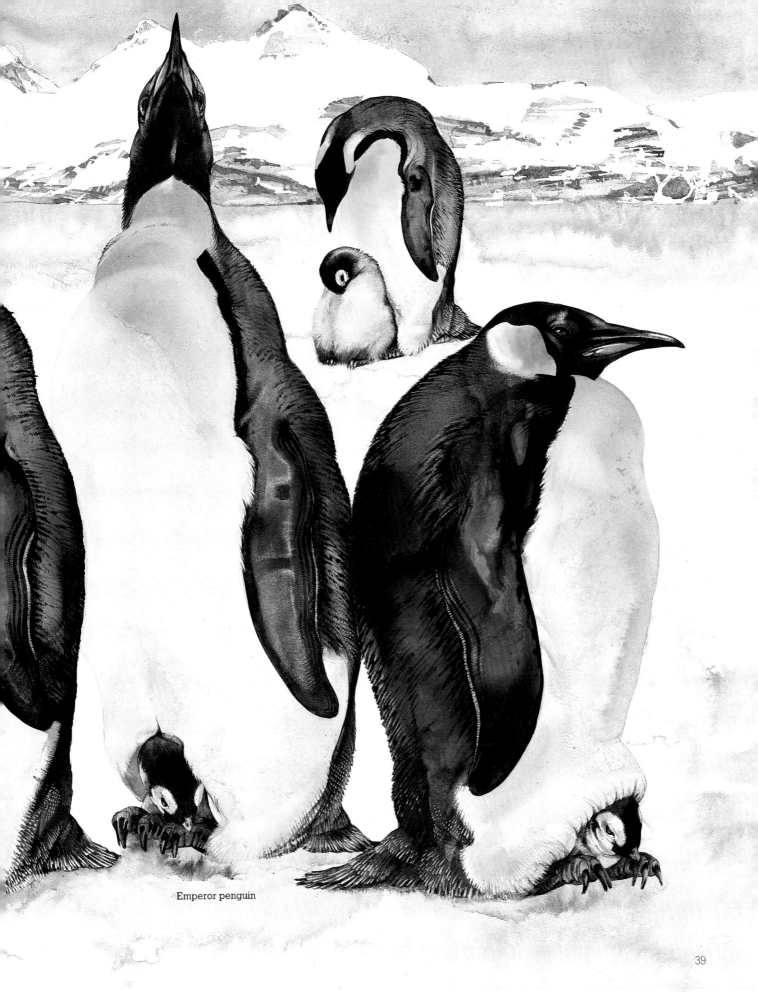

Emperor penguin

All the changes

In nine months in your mother's womb, you are transformed from a minuscule speck of living matter to something many millions of times heavier – a newborn baby. You grow into a toddler, a child, a teenager, an adult. As you grow older, your body changes all the time. When you look at the face of someone very old, you see a sort of map of all the changes that person has been through. You will go through similar changes. It is as if, in your lifetime, you are wrapped in countless different bodies, for your body never stops changing from the first moment it is made.

The changes are not simply a matter of growing bigger – there are also changes of form, as a caterpillar becomes a butterfly or a tadpole becomes a frog. Your changes are not as dramatic as these, but even so a baby enlarged to adult size would look nothing like an adult. Some of the most striking changes take place in adolescence, when a boy's body is becoming a man's and a girl's a woman's. These changes prepare your body for reproduction, the adult act of taking care of the future.

Human beings can choose whether or not to have babies, as no other animal can; but they cannot choose whether or not to die. It makes sense that we do not live for ever, however sad individual deaths may be. If dying had not been a fact of life from the beginning, the first living cells from 4,000 million years ago would still be here today – and all the great variety of beautiful bodies on earth would never have evolved. You were born because of all the lives which went before you, and because of all the changes which happened through time.

Your body is made from chemicals, which live and grow and change and enjoy all the wonders and adventures of the earth. Eventually you return to your quiet starting point. You are a baby, a child, an adult. You live, you eat and drink, you reproduce, you die. You belong to yesterday and tomorrow as surely as you belong to today. For the processes of life begin over and over again.

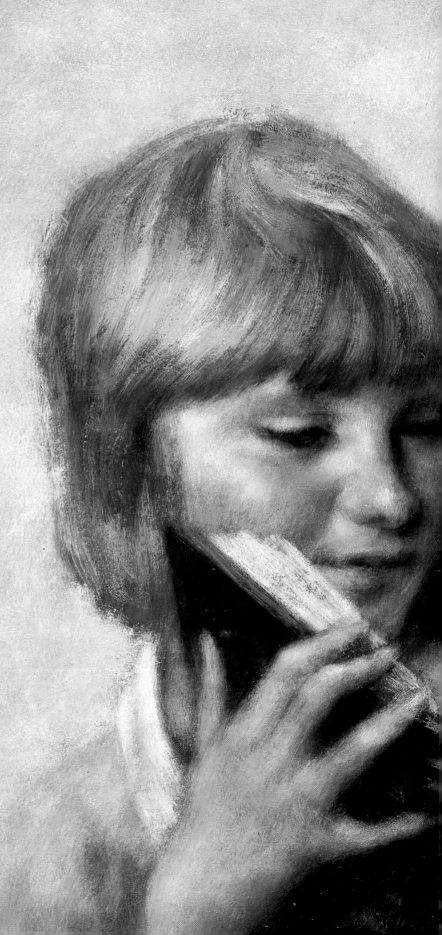

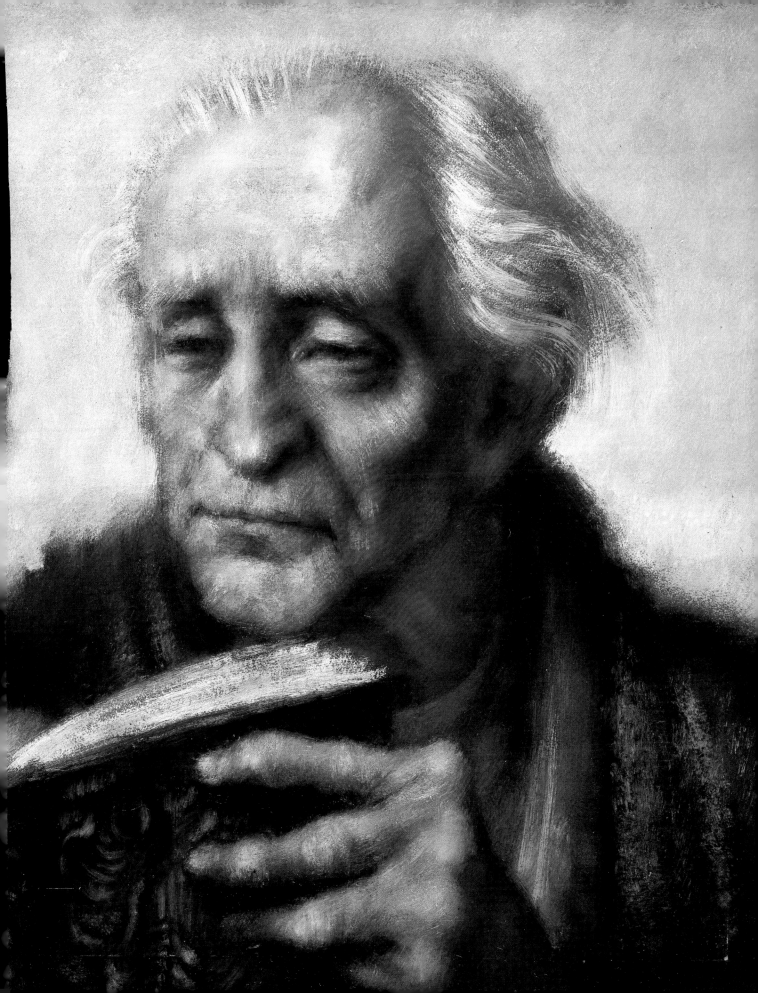

One hand clapping

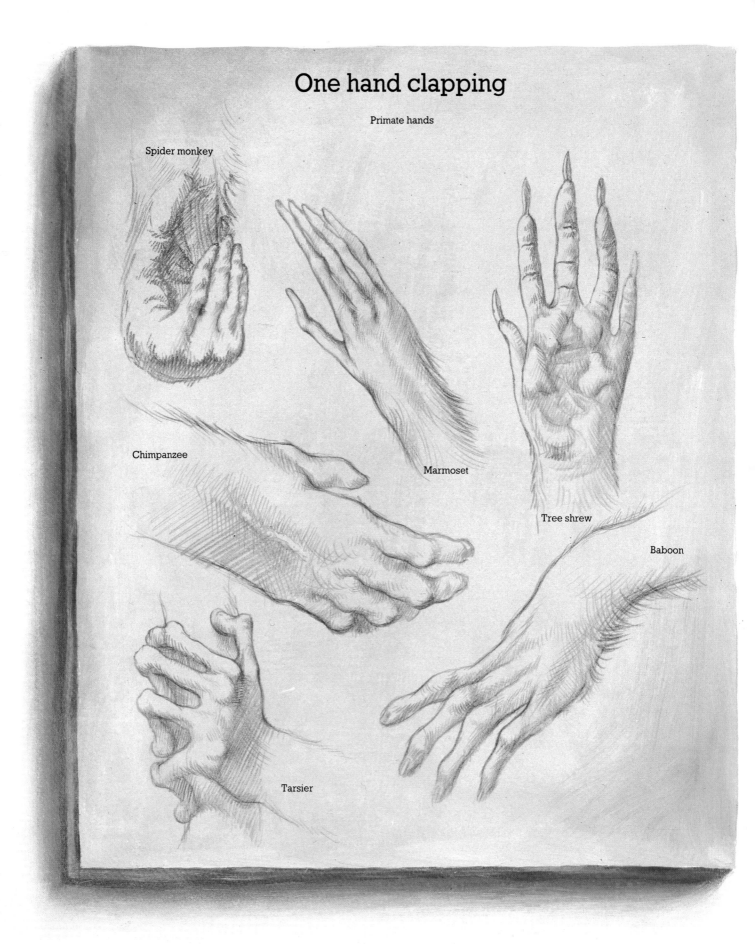

Primate hands

Spider monkey

Marmoset

Tree shrew

Chimpanzee

Baboon

Tarsier

The beauty of a body is not so much what it looks like as how it works. The beauty of a flamingo is its filter beak, its long legs for wading, its feathers – everything about it which adapts it to survive. The beauty of a dandelion or an elephant is the same – a matter of adaptation. You may say that one plant or animal looks more beautiful than another; but this beauty exists only in your eye, and in the judgement of your brain. In the wholeness of nature – where there is no judgement, but only survival through adaptation – all bodies are equal in their beauty.

The human body, your body, takes its place among all the others, and at first sight there is nothing very special about it. Other bodies see better, hear better, run better, swim better – do almost everything better, in fact, or do things which you cannot do at all, like fly. But no other body can do so much as yours with its hands, or imagine so many things for hands to do.

Imagining is a capacity of the brain, and the human brain is the most highly evolved in the world. The brains and hands of other living primates – your nearest animal relatives – are less advanced. They work perfectly in the context of these animals' lives, but they would not work in yours. You are a very brainy animal, with clever hands. This is the beginning of what makes you special.

By the power of thought, and skill at making things, human beings overcome the limitations of their bodies. They fly in planes, swim across oceans in boats, run about in cars, see far into the universe with telescopes. They even overcome the limitations of their brains, storing memories in books, for instance. By hand someone makes a brush, and with the brush you paint a dandelion. By hand you copy and applaud the wonder of the world.

More than all this, you can judge between good and evil, right and wrong, beautiful and ugly. This is the privilege and pleasure of being human. It is also a great responsibility. For the immediate well-being of life on earth, and the continuing existence of all this beauty, now depends on human decisions and actions.

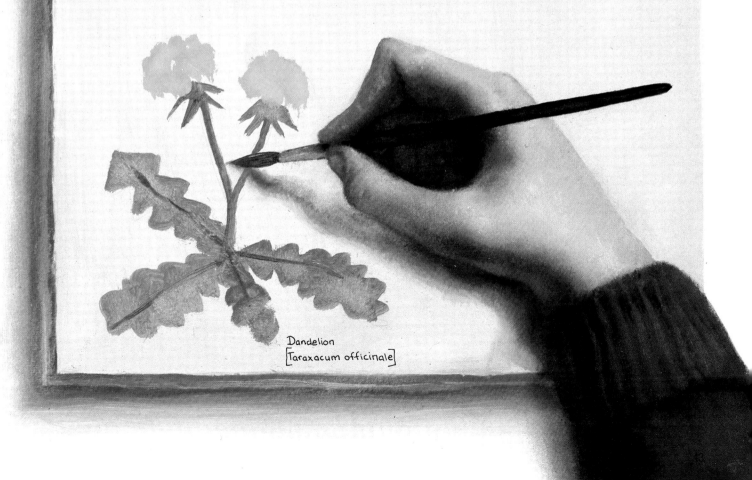

Dandelion
[Taraxacum officinale]

Index

Words in *italic* are Latin names of species noted in this book. Numbers in *italic* indicate illustrations.

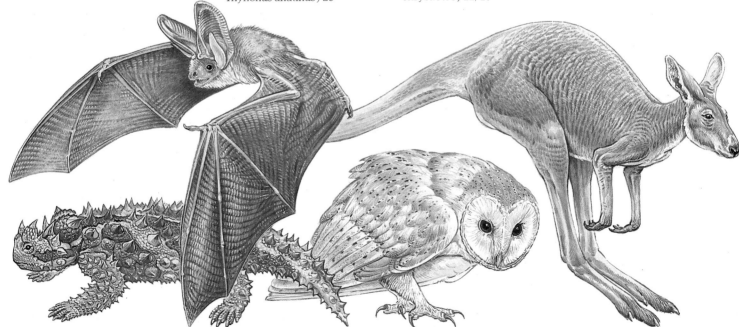

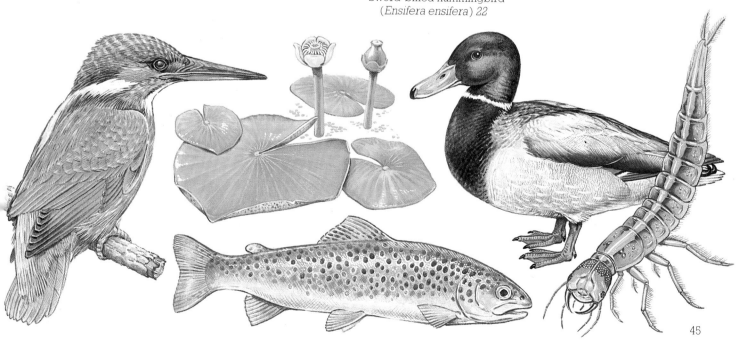

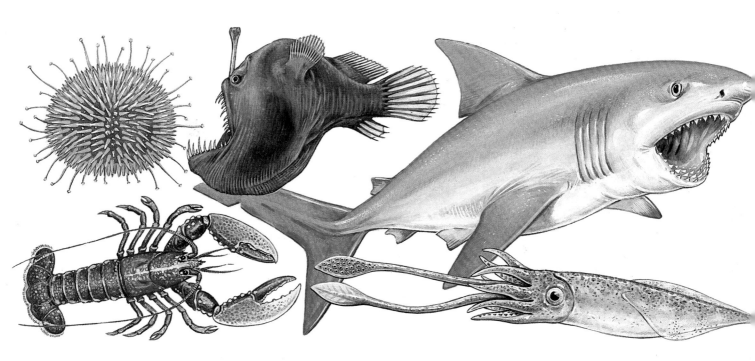